Paper Boat

Paper Boat
Poems

Cullen Bailey Burns

Cullen Bailey Burns

For Angie —
you are a treasured
friend.
love
Cullen

n
e
w
RIVERS
PRESS
MSUM

Library of Congress Card Catalog Number: 00-109782
ISBN: 0-89823-213-9
Minnesota Voices Project #101, 2003
Cover design by Percolator. Interior designed by Renae Brandner.

Printed in Canada

The publication of *Paper Boat* has been made possible by generous grants from the Jerome Foundation, Dayton's Project Imagine with support from the Target Foundation, and the Elmer L. and Eleanor J. Andersen Foundation.

This activity is made possible, in part, by a grant provided by the Minnesota State Arts Board, through an appropriation by the Minnesota State Legislature. In addition, this activity is supported, in part, by a grant from the National Endowment for the Arts.

Additional support has been provided by the General Mills Foundation, the McKnight Foundation, the Star Tribune Foundation, and the contributing members of New Rivers Press.

New Rivers Press is a nonprofit literary press associated with Minnesota State University Moorhead.

Wayne Gudmundson, *Director*
Alan Davis, *Senior Editor*
   Part-time Managing Editor: Donna Carlson
   Work Study: Charane Wilson
   Honors Apprentice: Robyn Schuricht
   Development intern: Sandra Arnau-Dewar
   Editorial interns: Kristen Garaas-Johnson, Athena Gracyk, Bret Hoveskeland, Crystal Jensen, Jessie Johnson, Anna Klein, Leslie Knudson, Carrie Olofson, Brett Ortlet, Josh Smith, Kristen Tsetsi
Julie Mader-Meersman, *Design and Production Director*
   Design Assistants: Erin Bieri, Renae Brandner, Shannon Tomac
   Photography Assistant: Rachel Broer
   Web Site Development: Daniel Norby (2002), Timothy Litt (2003)
   MSUM Student Technology Team: John Jeppson, Bo Vargas
Susan Geib, *Marketing Director*
   Marketing Manager: Karen Engelter
Nancy Edmonds Hanson, *Promotions Manager*
Marlane Sanderson, *Business Manager*
   Assistant Business Manager: Andy Peeters

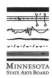

New Rivers Press
c/o MSUM
1104 7th Ave S.
Moorhead, MN 56563
www.newriverspress.com

For Michael Burns

and in memory of
Caitlin Bailey
1967-1994

Contents

Grateful acknowledgment is made to the following publications where some of these poems first appeared, sometimes in different versions.

Commitas: "The Hem of her Skirt," "Painting to Hold Emily"
Gulf Coast: "The Last Word"
Hayden's Ferry Review: "Hunting Trip, T. Bailey, 1929"
Laurel Review: "In Raspberries"
Luna: "Falling In"
Passages North: "Milk Money," "To War and Arms," "In the World"
Poetry Northwest: "Contrition"
Sonora Review: "Sight Words"
Walking Papers: "About its Task," "Autumnal"

Special thanks to the Minnesota State Arts Board for a generous fellowship that allowed me time to work on these poems. Thanks also to Norcroft: A Writing Retreat for Women, where many of these poems were written. I am grateful, too, to the support of Kathleen Mcgookey, David Dodd Lee, and Beth Roberts for their help and encouragement and wisdom.

Whither should my heart flee from my heart?
—St. Augustine

Your voice is gone now; I hardly hear you
Your starry voice all shadow now
—Louise Gluck

The Hem of Her Skirt

Here is no great measure – not begin,
not end – a simple sugar of now, one second
exploding. At the depot of the past
my sister wears jewelry, each piece
a different story, but at this morning's station
 – a handful of tarnished necklaces
from the back of my bureau drawer –
the faintest perfume rises.

And then in the dim fall light, green
finally frozen from the impatiens,
direction fails me. Back to the beginning
of memory, the continuous present tense?
The heart, harbinger of bright hopes,
views a whole life every second,
every beat, the just now, just now
hem of her skirt, stone of her necklace,
wave of her hand,
words long gone.

The Word for Building Her Back

What I mean to say,
as the rain falls through the reddening leaves,
is what I move my mouth against:
a wafer could be Christ, words could build her,
bit by bit, back into flesh. Can I get this right?
This once? To say I don't mean grief
though the words fall that direction, like petals,
like pearls. There is a delight
in the wrong thing, bad manners, the older sister
always getting it wrong. If I could find
the silent spot in the middle of each minute
maybe the longing would cease. I mean
that rain falling sound, how it matches a good kiss
in full sun, how it rhymes with every sad word
then one by one refutes each. Toads and pearls,
toads and pearls; I'm settling for that one zinnia,
fat as a heart, signifying an enduring, slipshod joy.

On Memory

1

The past is like that

gesture – hands lifted
a certain way to a mouth:

a shimmy, a twitch above water,
line invisible

and we don't know the half of it.

To be drawn in,
walleye, catfish

girl walking a high wall
and saying she remembers.

2

This is what you must say: Ronald McDonald McDonald make a
      biscuit.
How do you like my love. A biscuit. He's so fine.
Just like a bottle of wine. A biscuit.
Now clap: together. Again. Again.
Until you can be as fast with me as she was, until our
      hands itch and tingle and we clap,
until we are two girls in a U Haul, our father driving west
      through Pennsylvania.
So follow the rules, chin up, and I'll make a sister of you
      yet.

3

This morning after the first hard frost
geraniums and tomatoes lay down their reds
for winter.
In the blue, cold sky the geese
go warmth-ward
and whatever those black birds are
that fly together like one long bolt of silk

unfurled across the sky
pass over the airport
for hours.
Lovely. Be mine.

4
A man and two girls fish for walleye
in 1977. Northern Michigan, a lake
called Opal, diamonds of light
in their eyes. *Sunfish, sunfish* one girl
calls out who has died since and left me
to remember.

Autumnal

See the auspicious world with its monarchs
and milkweed, geese calling *winter*
to the turning leaves of fall. See
the lake chock full of herons
bulking up for the long flight south.
See the magic of our hearts
burst or tire after life astonishes
one last time. What's known
is as much as anything,
the eclipsed moon in earth's shadow,
what we say *all* to, what
we say *there* to, what we learn
returns to a yard, to an evening,
to one in-drawn breath:
hope and bright stars aiming down.

Feast of the Holy Innocents

Child with your head that aches
week to week, that one lobe
confounding the others with its patterns
like lightning,
you were born on the calendar's unluckiest day.

Nights when you curl into your body
and your pain, your skin damp,
all your girl energy given to hurt,
I think of those children mistaken
for Christ,
the many deaths worked out for them.

As if an idea could comfort parents –
their baby forever companion to Jesus.
But you of the wild hair and thin legs,
you whom language mystifies
and trips,
the full cup's measure of your life

couldn't relieve me of you,
even into the arms of God.

Fall as a Kiss

Fall is more than a long descent,
giggly darling, kidnapper,
upon whose lips *maybe*
beautifies. Scrutinize as the wind
does, trees bent down before it,
I do, your arms like feathers,
like shackles, me here, sky
everywhere. Fall and you on the other side
of possible, what is meant by *there*.
Teeth and skin and language,
strange brew of fates.
Future, gainsayer, what will be

made of this: the lake hopeful against the sky,
every lie like sugar on my lips?

On Longing

In the snow that fell last night, fine dust,
a trail of stepped-on pomegranate seeds
purple the steps of Clara Barton School.
Ten days before Christmas, a woman walking to her
        daughter's room
thinks of Demeter and her six unbearable months,
of daughters with their shoulders and morning glories,
their ever-changing mouths turned to the whole world,
what they can get of it, what yields.
A girl can disappear.
A mother, over the rubbed bones of a goat,
her wrists wound in white string, will do what the shaman
says. The blood of three chickens and the yolk
of three eggs mixed in a wooden bowl. Your girl
will come back. A girl can disappear.
Wind chill already 15 below, live things dug in
till the thaw comes, union of need and mothering (see
all the dresses the mother's pressed for her?
the clipped articles to be read?).
One mother freezing the world
to match her heart and all the rest hoping magic
or love or stepping carefully
across a frozen, ruby-colored mess
will keep the girl, keep her out
of harm's way.

Indictment

You say Miner Lake has frozen again after the unseasonable
    thaw,
holes for fishing drilled back in
with precision. And the long days

of children keep you inside. I did not
tell you it would be so –
Barbie's work boots tiptoeing

endlessly through days
when time expands

and contracts
and there will never be enough
I am telling you now. But see,

you are caught up again in two small hands
inside your own, shoe strings held loosely,
girl on your lap: loop and wrap, push through and pull.

On the lake a man pulls a blue gill through a round hole in
    ice,
drops it down into the snow, a beautiful death,
the sun shines weakly,

and you, you are writing none of this down.

Counting

The girl in the red chair has not brushed her hair.
She leans against the arm rest with her legs pulled up
making a small *a* of her body. She holds
a silver cake server in her hand,
turns it to catch and throw the light against the wall,
against the cat. Her hair is a brownish jumble
of dreams of bees and money, and her bare legs
are prickled with goosebumps,
but she doesn't notice, chin on her knees,
eyes watching the light dance. Christmas in six
days and the snow all ruined by rain. The girl
matches things up: chair to poinsettia,
coffee table to Christmas tree trunk. She counts
to ten over and over, to click time off
on this hard wait and when she gets to seven
sometimes she stops and says, "I'm seven,
I'm seven, I'm seven years old,"
flashing the magic silver in her hands.

Maluco Beleza

The tree is up, brought all the way from
Michigan, because the land is in us

and ours is that vast peninsula;
ours is risen out of water,

the rough-edged world,
cliffs and boats going down.

Lakes that tell the whole story: boys and fish
and violence and all the sex

that happens near water. So we say
we live *heart-to-the-wind*

ears tuned to a pitch
just this side of hearing.

We say so. Trimmed, then, in light, the tree:
we take *home* with us. We will.

On My Sister's Ascension to Heaven

1
The valkyries, with their kind, strong arms
swoop down

and bear up
the body, beloved,
unclothed, bear up the body.

2
The white light
bright heart
a pull toward happy
and stepping there
this world falls away.
Light and all
but not easy, maybe,
to let the lived life drop.

3
Build a tree house,
build a pyre,
ashes making their way up.
Skin ash, bone ash, hair ash,
eye ash, lip ash, lung ash. The finest
particles given to wind, given back to earth
in the end.

4
There is no heaven,
and she is simply gone. Today
the air was so many degrees below zero
it buckled the streets and starters of buses,
cast everybody back indoors. A still minute broken by a
        laugh,
exhaust cartwheeling from tailpipes.
There is no heaven maybe, but this sky at dusk
dyeing the snow blue and lighting it from within
is a kind of everlasting with her in it.

Contrition

What is there to regret?...if I had to be born a thousand times again,
I would be a thousand times what I have been.
—Klaus Barbie

He had to say that. See how the leaves have yellowed and begun to clutter
the sidewalk like something important parked behind the car, like Maggie's
trike. A logical place to park, really, until I pulled *A.J.Foyt backs out of the
driveway* and can't apologize enough. But he couldn't say you children can't
possibly understand what I'm about to do. Better to take it as a job well done.
My girl never stepping in the path of a car, say, or hating me someday for
ways I've erred. And I have, oh, taken her perfect arms and said *you must put
this shirt on*, or *I'm gonna swat your butt*, or *why are you so goddamned stub-
born*. And ten million apologies won't change my carelessness, my hair-into-
the-wind stomp on the accelerator, pushing the bike all sideways on itself,
that tiny metal crunch. She might have been on it. And whose children were
they, rolling off to camps with names like china breaking – Treblinka, Bergen
Belsen, Dachau; children waiting for their big teeth to grow in. He had to say
he'd do it again. No other life could forgive him.

Afternoon Light, January

You know this field, snow covered, corn stalks
bent down from the combines, a man
at the far side ringing a bell.
He means come or danger or help
but you can't be sure in this light
leaning its yellow across land, giving winter
its due. It's palpable, the light;
not warm but taken in like air.
And noise winds out, clapper
to silence,

rumbles up from the deep spots
in our hearts where arteries tear
or balloon, where we keep secrets
the surgeons see when they spread
the embracing ribs.
What could we know about
the old contraption pounding us along?

And you know me, how I've taken
to my bed, tired of words and things
trying to match themselves up.
Better this:

January light angled across the floor,
a yellow cat in the warm spot, and
a clock clicking its hands across time.
Better tea and a pet and a sky wide open
and a rug for girls to watch spin
after they've twirled themselves
into dizziness. Listen how the past
rattles its bones until they sound like words –
if I could say it comes to this

we'd be no closer to it,
heart, dear heart.

One Sure Thing

Stepping back,
bearing her voice and skin with her,
who cartwheeled past the Washington Monument

with a cigarette in one hand:
my sister. Now sun pools on the floor,
a warm spot cross-hatched

by panes, shadows of panes,
but when I sit here my back
can't feel the places

the sun isn't. January and the snow
leaves its pictures in my eyes
long after I look away.

I try to remember
this day's light on this day's floor,
a voice

I never thought about.
Now will nothing be sure again:

had and lost
and longed for –
constellation bearing down from each new sky?

Story

A rock-a-bye.
A rock-a-bye.
A cardinal on the sill.

Ice and water, ice and water,
a little bit of winter on the lake.

I will tell a story called again:
last year's volunteer tomatoes,
what our milky mouths once asked the world;
I will tell of sky, cloudless,
of equinox.

Once there was a man
who lifted (heavy work) a salmon
from silver water. See,
love makes girls out of fish,
possibility, legs and hair and face
grown from a salmon. She danced
in thunder, years passed.
He watched and watched,
fed her oysters and milk.
Love created fragile
grown-long bones of a daughter,
this seen, held and raised up girl,
but not his he learns, watching her
skin throwing light like scales,
not really and not safe.
So he throws her back
lies alone on the bluffs:
had I known.

The ice will melt.
The one loon will rest the one night and one day
she always does on Diamond Lake, on her way
to some place from another.
The earth will lean us closer to the sun.
The heart

– like a robin, not subtle, not lovely –
returns to loving, despite.

Sleep.

Helen and the First Grade

There is often a woman beneath the swan
white and vanishing, her whole self pulled
beyond touch.
Lies or a few obscuring clouds
testify simple against the multichambered heart.

There is often a child boarding a bus in the rain
that falls through sun and spells out a kiss, blown
from a girl's palm to air. Nothing
can stop the dog from growling at the bus
that takes his girl away.

There is often that swan and time
leaving its grip marks on a women's wrists.
The despised, done and undone,
gives way. And what is left is always a yellow bus,
and always pulling away.

To War and Arms

There was a woman and there was a war.
And the chance was upon him finally to say, "I could
not love thee dear so much, loved I not honor more."
But the woman rolled over in bed and wouldn't
be comforted. And the wind blew. And he saw
himself peeled back from his life like something
raw or rancid, what we tighten our skin around.
The war, as always, raged. The sky bruised. March,
mid-thirties most days. He took up smoking, leaning
against doorways, working on the look: noncommittal.
Finally she said I will not have soldiers in my house.
She lay on top of him one last time, light and solid,
and he carried her with him like a stone.
There was a woman and then a war.

Little Bit Snowing Song

Doesn't amount to much though it bevels the sky
with possibility.
But look here: a raincoat so small
what was can't possibly fit inside.
Snow falls like a half worked-out idea,
though the children aren't dressed for it
and it should have been rain.
Growing is effortless,
sipping tea,
never thinking this could be lost to me
or you could be lost
or the funny thing we call our love.
We keep changing this story
except for the facts: too little snow
to accumulate, bags of our old clothes
awaiting the Salvation Army,
the Christmas cactus in bloom all year
and our children always past the place
in time we reach for them.

Success

There is always this business of possibility,
what the long married see in each other –
less of this, more of that, and the rhubarb
they planted when they began still burrowing
out of winter and into pie. Not love, exactly,
but a life, smaller than a half dollar fallen
right out of a body and held in a palm.
Or the business of enough. Success.
Another good meal. -50 wind-chill last night
but la la la la warm house, coffee steaming, a man
desiring the all of me. I can't think, winter pressing
the blue sky, sunlight pure and steady, down. An eggplant
on the counter, two onions. We will make dinner
of this. We'll make of the bits enough to go on,
awed and sated. Love, build a fire. I am afraid.

Clean Sweep

A solitary man practices his jump shot,
pushing into the left-footed leap,
and the world contracts into that ball
brushing the backboard like a kiss –
but I'm the driver of the blue car
he doesn't see, and my glimpse of him
is of every man I've ever watched practicing.
I've spent days sweeping the ceiling for cobwebs
hanging in every corner. And if all things
move toward chaos, what do I make of the right arm
arcing to the bent-down rim?
Some mornings breakfast is enough to make me
put my head down and sing a Janis Joplin song, the fact
that I'm older now than she ever was adding
just a bit of her gravel to my voice. My POW bracelet
is buried in Girl Scout Troop 31's time capsule
under a tree in Crane Park. And my POW is probably
beneath the mud in Vietnam. I gave the bracelet
emblematically to my troop leader and tried to cry.
When I remember my POW, but not his name, it's in the same
        casual way
the fuzzy men on tv bounded on the moon
while my mother said, "be quiet. Someday it will be
        important you watched this."
Her cigarette smoke patterning the room. In fourth grade
        every noon I'd walk home
for lunch and eat alone,
while my mom ironed to the words
of Haldeman or Sirica, occasionally damning the iron.
Even now I can't separate anger and cleanliness. Sweep
        floors, walls ceilings,
vacuum furniture, blinds, impeachment, war. Gangs of
        neighborhood boys
spiraling footballs across the playground
and spitting and calling what's-his-name a pussy. I'd drag
        my toes across the sand
while I sat in my metronome swing, watching.
Sometimes one boy would tackle me

and we'd fall in a nice-feeling pile
until I'd scream for him to get up.
Things I didn't know
I suspected, like the man in the car who asked me
wanna see me jack off?
and embarrassed me just by the look on his face.
Now almost everyday some errand sends me past my buried
POW bracelet and the men who park their cars
beside the trees and wait – longings I understand even less
than how to spin the stitches on the football
from my fingertips, or how to three step it
to the basket, a clean sweep, the basketball
rolling itself from my hand.

Lake Memory

Cold again and rain falls
on the needleless Christmas tree at the curb,
the tipped geraniums. Cold again:
this spring's been a test of heavy skies.
Sirens pulse by in drizzle –
someone else's calamity.

There have been hours
when Lake Michigan became all waves
I'd crest and ride above the undertow.
Not quite summer but the lake's there,
and there's certain comfort in that.
In February I stood on mountains the lake made,
ice bridges into the slow moving water.
So much heft and the cracklings
of force and resistance.

Even on this side of spring, trilliums three petals
are what we need some days.
Once I thought I saw Jesus climb a chainlink fence
and walk toward me. What could I have told
to such a face as that? On another lake
the sandhill crane cocked its head
and froze into a rush or cattail, still in the shade
cast from a quick-moving cloud.
It stood and stood, waiting for me to stop seeing,
to move into the world of breathing creatures.
The peat buzzes and sometimes uncovers people with their
stories
in their pockets – flint and seeds. The gnats
and dragonflies rise up like ash,
drone our names over and over.
In the world that already knows how this story's told
I sometimes can't stand up
to memory's snap in my brain.
My girls run ahead
in wild geranium, hepatica, oak saplings
no thicker than their wrists,

into the dunes where we make
a family of held hands and leap
almost past gravity, gut laughing our way down.

Dispossession

I've looked in the grass and under bark the woodpecker's
      pulled back.
I've looked for signs
in the way light falls across
a morning, something besides
goldfinches in thimbleberries, seagulls bobbing
like buoys on the lake.

Superior has said:
      you expect what?
      Crying lady name my colors;
      name your heart
      in words I can understand.

      Lie on black rocks
      steaming water to air
      and see how easily

      I relinquish that which was never mine
      and is myself.

Birthday, Girl

And then you were with me
like an arrowhead just uncovered in the back yard,
a terra-cotta soldier.
There was no doubt,
never even a second, it seemed,
that you hadn't changed.
Passion is my story
though your body will become fire
and dazzle soon. We attest this,
each to the other. Now chalk and lilacs,
a nest propped up in the Linden tree,
nest for a found robin's egg – you
slept your weight into my chest,
loveliest burden
from that first instant onward.

Painting to Hold Emily

Paint-thick waves and in the middle
a girl with a brown egg
in her left hand. Her long hair,
yellow, pulled back. She sits
on a stool, thinks of grass
and third grade and is still.
Fish – butterfly, angel and bass –
swim the red waves.
Milk in her blue cup
and hours could go fast or slow,
depending. And years could go fast or slow,
depending. And she could grow or not,
even set the egg on the stool and swim away,
depending.

On Flight

What I thought I saw:
the pumping of wings,
the hard work of ascension –
for the broad-winged and delicate
heron, egret, the up and down,
the undulation, legs trailing,
an after-thought.
I was mistaken.
It was a man. Flying.
His wheelchair soared
the paved shoulder of the hill,
his arms rose and fell,
swooped and lifted,
wings, from a distance,
flight, from a distance:
two things at once he was then
for perceiver and, perhaps, perceived.

Milk Money

There are days when everyone
is reaching for the ground.
The chicken restaurant in my town says
only one life, twill soon be past
only what's done for Christ will last
on every twelve piece bucket.

I have thought about this, because
on Sesame Street one morning was a chicken factory
where chicks hatched beneath lights,
dropped to belts and circuited through gloved hands
that separated boys from girls,
put them in the proper cages, where the film ended –
happy chicks pecking their grain.

My kids say, "Can we get real chicks for Easter?"
and I see my mother shudder, telling how the chicken's head
flopped in the yard after the axe came down,
forty years making her story only bloodier, epic.

The wind has lost its edge and I walk the girls to school.
They run ahead, feeling spring as they feel sadness,
sudden and intuitive. The ground loosens, trees bud,
and tonight the family rises up in hunger saying
please more chicken. Jesus must be somewhere

bending down a little, looking for the milk money
that always slips through envelopes
the children carry with them to school.

Cup to Moon

Listen, Black-eyed Susans mean the world
to me. Beneath crickets and Queen Anne's Lace
dirt smells of the body
and the world speaks.

Children fall into sewers, are bashed
into walls by their parents.
Me, I drink mine down to leaves
in the bottom of a cup

then spread them beneath
velvet and protecting eyes
in the far field of wild flowers
and danger.
Which becomes the future.

Which is why my mother gave me
a success agenda
to measure days to rhythm
and accordance. In this way
the unexpected –

So if we don't move,
yellow-pealed, black-hearted Susans and I,

or breathe too much,
I can invent the world and children
safe from my palm to damp earth,
cup to moon,
and frost when it comes
so soon.

Evocation at Dusk

Bee neck-deep in the purple thistle,
soft part for touching or diving into,
thistle plant taller than a pretty tall woman,
taller than that. If deer should come,
finally, to the trees and a downward slant
of land, could they be real deer? Or just hoped
for among the hummocks in the tall grass,
their declivities. And if the deer pull leaves
from the small trees near the window,
so that their eyes reflect a window with a woman
on the other side drinking ginger tea with lemon, then
must they be flesh and hair and ticks? Twitches
on their hides? The nervous half-lifted
rear foot, hindquarter shuddering off flies?
If the sun makes spots of air warmer, where
it lands through balsams and birch, could
it be a good evening for deer, even though
the lake's disappeared into haze? Real
deer, with round eyes and a white flap
of tail, this incantation to draw you,
a summons, goes out and out into evening.

Letter to My Mother

It is the art of a minute:
phlox in a green vase,
the Venus di Milo song you used to sing

in the days that disappear now,
very slowly, and what's left: our hands
dusted with moth wing glister.

Today men came and fixed my water
that you worried over, and the heavy-
headed peonies have blossomed.

What you asked was same,
a comfort, a wing.
The Japanese kimono specifically

for a woman tortured by demons. We know distress
can be a kind of beauty – red or white, gold foil
adhered to silk, called surihaku.

Behind the glass in the museum
(No costume, Middle Edo period, eighteenth century)
it shimmers like the part it played,

but we are women
of small perfections. We sang in the car
for hours, I curled into your lap for years

and the world flashed.
The robe is plain beside
the blues and reds and plum blossoms

the open fans and butterflies,
what the world might be to noblemen
and soldiers. What the world might be

to slip inside and tell:
goodbye the demons mumble
into our ears.

How silk deepens in certain light,
becomes the sky where last night stars were gold
and, mother, I could touch.

Blue Earth

Probably in July, the corn asserting its green stalks as summer,
she gave the baby up. Might not even have dressed it,
besides a diaper and the one soft blanket. Probably
she was too young or too old with many other mouths
making their red demands. Could even be he hit her,
or loved her so she was always saying yes.

But it happened, at least, in Blue Earth,
flat-edged Minnesota, where rows and rows
of corn rose up one summer of enough rain,
enough sun and not too many grasshoppers.
At night wolves and foxes stole chickens. And in winter
when the stars settled so close to rooftops the roofs

might blaze, air twenty or thirty below, the girl
melted frost from the window with the small circle
of her mouth and began her story,
one she would tell until the last years of the century.
And it began: My real mother...

Hunting Trip, 1929, T. Bailey

Mountains in the background like bad props –
California or the badlands –
and a man front and center
with high boots and a rifle
and a satisfied smile. It's 1929.
He's got nothing to lose
in the stock market and a deer slug
like the world across his shoulders.
A deer held by its ear, head
cradled beneath the man's chin.
And while it looks as if the man
could whisper anything into that ear,
bounty or the saga of the hunt,
it is the deer, eyes staring through
sixty years, planets, unchanging,
suggesting the uncle's too many drinks
and then the suicide, suggesting
this is a photo of who whispers to whom.

Loss Said:

before me all was perfection,
trees bore fruit, flowers opened their pretty mouths
to God. But who could see

in this profusion?
Air so sweet and perfect lawns that bade you
lie hours and hours not recognizing contentment.

In some ways I am your gift.
See, see
the apple tree still blossoms pink
but how articulate against
an absolute blue sky.
And remember how you stopped,

breath drawn in,
beauty taking pain's place
in your body?

Still you resist me. You think
in staring hours at the floor
I'll turn out to have come to the wrong house?
No, I've come and gone,

taking your dear one with me
so you could see

July. Beauty. The inescapable
felt world.
And now you must.

In Raspberries

Before the children wake to wet air, 80s,
July inching its way toward fall, before
cereal is poured into blue bowls, topped
with milk and fighting begins over who reads
the box first, before even the garbage
truck grinds the rest of the way through the alley,
will be a moment, robin and jay filled, when a woman
bends over berry bushes, gathering fruit
for breakfast or for the fact of solitude:
hundreds of tiny hearts in a plastic bucket asking
something of this world.

Ravishing

I've been a woman heavy
      on the lee side of love
all hips and ravishes. There is no
      surviving the onslaught.

I've seen the night sky toss
      its satellites across a man's back,
the crickets a Greek chorus
      chanting *you will be disappointed; there is a hard*
          fate
awaiting you. But hell, what do crickets know.

Except fate is always hard,
      whether it be drought
or the shimmer of 105 rising off the corn. What do
      crickets know, singing summer along,
except the heart too can shimmer
      as it burns.

For All the World

Heavy rain has tilted the cosmos and pansies,
bowed them headlong to the ground. Except the zinnias,
orange no less, looking straight into the cloud swept sky.

This is a scrap of paper; this is another day.
With rain or without. With a half-moon
of a garden or without. Listen, none of this matters –
not the way we held our daughters' hands and leapt
down Sleeping Bear Dunes, bounding bounding
through gravity and sun,
not the muskie restless in the warming lakes of July –
without a mouth to give in to,
a lake to take the place of the future,
a you to right me in this wind,

you with your arms and patience, holding me up for all the
        world.

Before the Lake

Suppose I were to tell you I am a woman in need of consoling. Suppose I were to tell you I am not. Lake Superior breaks and breaks against these iron colored rocks. And then: a heart, a heart or disbelief. Suppose a letter arrived with news of home, that distance. Instead, an envelope carrying nothing, good words lost across the state. Suppose a woman walked down to water. There, above the lake cold as love or December, she lifted her face to the sky. But perhaps the sky, wide as the lake and as gray, provided her a sadness so acute she couldn't move. Like Niobe who begged fate then lost her fourteen children to her pride, the woman could turn stone. For suppose I am that woman and the lake's inexorable forth and back, articulate and ancient beneath me, helps me think: I have, I have. But an empty envelope and my dear ones truly lost, forth and back, waves, suppose I displeased and my loves were lifted from this indifferent and breathtaking world. Then could it be in that dark red sea of beginning inside me it is possible, still, the having. No matter the having to let go.

About Its Task

The earth erases,
no matter our ministrations.

When I call out aster, clover,
spotted-touch-me-not,

when I say clasping-leaved mullein,
lupine, yarrow,

the world is unchanged. Flowers have nothing
to do with their naming

and might just as soon go
nameless about their task

of overgrowing the path,
composing to their own cadence

and decomposing in time.
Adam, when he handed out the names,

believed in order. But the named things,
unhearing, mute, grew and died, healed

or injured their namer, as was their appointment.
This would have happened regardless

of a voice calling to morning:
bellflower, buttercup, birdsfoot trefoil,

red pine, water, rock.

In this World

Women might love like backhoes,
the sky be always blue.
Goldfinches on lovers' backs,
lighter than breath.
A man might ask a woman, "What's the definition of
    conduit?"
who answers correctly, turns him on.

The world of flimsy words: negligee, supple. Or here,
let's not say anything about the sky
resting like good intentions on our foreheads.
What's a backhoe do but dig earth,
tamp it down? And some men,

when they touched me, finally, words flew
and my body remembered every accidental shock,
its own surprised oh.
We return to the ground, beneath the mourning dove's
"do it, do, do, do,"
which sounds like a man
blowing air through cupped hands to make that low call.
We are buried in the hopes of rising up,
but listen, loves,

all of you: a minor rhapsody.

Fragment

and in the long future of plastic
this bottle to my lips
this comb through my daughter's hair
will tell
cell or mote
the infinitesimal story of family

Not What Lasts, What Is

Clover, broken brown leaves, how the street smells in May after a rain, in this rendering. A dog and a cat and two long-legged girls, a man and a house that stays warm. A whole Minnesota sky in November, sky so blue it says my name to remind me we belong to each other. A taste for squash and its smooth beige skin, a cup of milk, a red pear. To lie in the grass in May, to stare at Lake Superior the whole month of August, to pull a child into my lap and rest my face on her warm, round head. Oh uncomfortable pillow, oh mutable world. The dog rages at the mailwoman, the leaves have fallen. A little snow, too, just the start of the long months of cold. But I know spring and its good intentions, know the dog's pure optimism. There is no making this stay, not with paint or words or even my mouth pressed against my man's, and no reason not to try.

Revision

Of course it all begins with the apple,
the necessary emblem, the perfect air
in the yard, coneflowers and pachysandra
and bees as big as silver dollars. There is no proof
but the story, mouth to ear, generation
to generation. But here, in August, apples
bending the thin stems of trees, sun
and cool breezes ushering Fall, I read
of footsteps fossilized beside an African lake,
a woman's print left in wet mud
as she went about the business of gathering
roots or water at the same moment in time
we began our great shame.
Beside her in the water, no snake.
At home no flawless man awaiting
her return. Instead he carved
stone into spearheads, brushed flies
from his shoulders, and danger asked more
than any one story of God.

The Last Word

The lake says write this
and gives me bad rhymes
and rhythms for marching,
what a lake can muster up
for poetry.
She says *what? those rocks?*
Nothing, honey, worth marking down
on paper. She's agreeable
today, unequivocal queen
of the moment.
Those gulls?
Truly stupid, completely without
imagination. I'm
cold and wide and old
as anything on earth.
Metaphor that.

Sight Words

1

Penelope weaves all day above the noisy suitors
only to pull the fine threads out all night.
So that loyalty becomes something to do with the fingers.

Odysseus might have learned this, too, but Calypso…

She doesn't linger on the details of hue and complement;
just her busy fingers, nights pulling the strands back,
any ritual to keep her body from recognizing

obsession.

2

I dreamed the birds lifted simultaneously
from the walnut tree just
as the black-haired woman unbuttoned her blouse.

The buttons were mother of pearl,
glinting like my first boyfriend's teeth,
something requiring my mouth.

I dreamed the birds' wings were shawls for mourning,
draping the thin arms of old women,
or shrouds for the old dead men.

Grant me the dead are selves
our selves release like skeet
we aim for.

In early morning, from this chair, I know the woods are
     peopled
with spirits moving like deer
in pink light.

If a neighbor takes his bow out,
it's because when we die our gift is those
black eyes that help us forget our lives.

We can forget, that's the guarantee.

3

But you know this. Sight words,
Emily says, are words you just know.
And transubstantiation becomes you,
nodding to Penelope's labor,

how the heroic deeds of women involve such fine hands.
Of course Joe over there,

sinking his hands into his pockets,
looks on from another angle. He's seen

one man kill another and says
the more room you take up in your body the better.

Penelope bores him.

4

You people keep letting me put words into your mouth,
even move your mouth to those perfect Os of recognition,

at this rate I could touch you anywhere.
Up down in out off on over under.

These are sight words,
        says Emily.
And opposites, I say.
And sight words, says Emily.

5

Every fall monarch glance against the pink zinnias,
a gaudy picture, orange and black and flowered,
and the critic in me eyes it all:
how hope resembles that migration, so many recognizable
        figures
moving toward home.

Falling In

Once a man came to haul boxes.
Said, "$125 for such heavy boxes." Said, "I gotta pay,
        too,
you know, I gotta pay too." I watched the deep holes
in his face because they were all I could see
in the garage full of rubbish – rags
and light bulbs and thousands and thousands
of milk cartons. The holes were round and deep
as if a cheek were thicker than just one
soft wall of flesh, as if bone would have been
less galling. Because there is all this falling in
not to be done, the many ways I want
to see the body. One summer
I swam almost every night, under a moon
in a little lake that had no name. I would
swim with one man or another, our bodies
another element out of water, air and fire.
Are there words for this?
For the transforming water
and the arms of a nineteen year old boy?
The ways we treaded slowly
above fish and duck weed and the silt of the years?
What does it mean to remember
sensation without language
to salve the intervening years? Some nights
when the neighbor pauses outside my house
to light his cigarette, his dog straining
at the leash, I am sure the red ember,
the exhaled smoke, are messages from the past
I can barely remember, except in bits, in the floating
my body does on its way into sleep, in a certain
touch – one man's hand through my hair –
or the breeze through an opened window
in June. The body breaks down and every year
reminds me of its inarticulate beauty, its
inexpressible keening.

I Have Made a Paper Boat

and set words aflame upon water,
a message the lake
carries to the dead.

Fire (on water,
fire) on the last element
she knew,

bid her safe passage.

A wave, a kiss,
water lays down
the path.

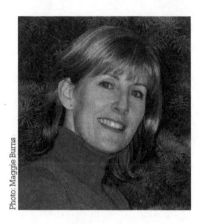

Photo: Maggie Burns

Cullen Bailey Burns lives in Minneapolis and teaches at Century College. She is a recipient of a 1999 Minnesota State Arts Board Artist Fellowship. Her poems have appeared in *Poetry Northwest, The Sonora Review, Hayden's Ferry Review, Luna* and others. A Michigan native, she received her MFA from Western Michigan University.